Sirtfood Diet

Recipes

Breakfast and Lunch

The Complete Guide to Burn Fat and Get Lean Muscle with Tasty and Easy Recipes

Laura Hamilton

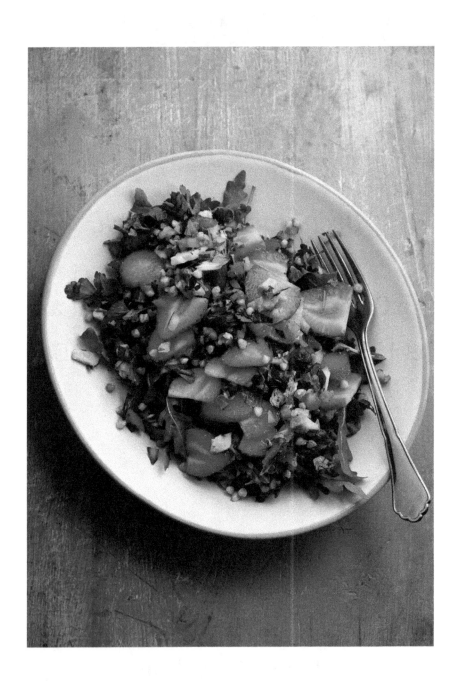

including specific information will be considered an illegal act irrespective of if it is done electronically or in print. This extends to creating a secondary or tertiary copy of the work or a recorded copy and is only allowed with the express written consent from the Publisher. All additional right reserved.

The information in the following pages is broadly considered a truthful and accurate account of facts and as such, any inattention, use, or misuse of the information in question by the reader will render any resulting actions solely under their purview. There are no scenarios in which the publisher or the original author of this work can be in any fashion deemed liable for any hardship or damages that may befall them after undertaking information described herein.

Additionally, the information in the following pages is intended only for informational purposes and should thus be thought of as universal. As befitting its nature, it is presented without assurance regarding its prolonged validity or interim quality. Trademarks that are mentioned are done without written consent and can in no way be considered an endorsement from the trademark holder.

Table of Contents

SirtFood Diet Explained

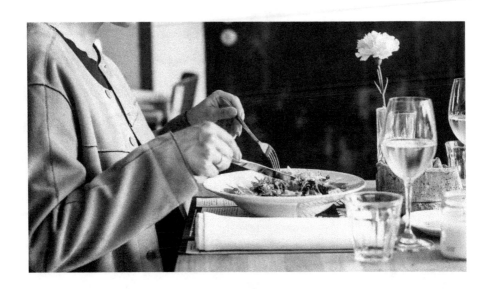

According to nutritionist Rob Hobson, Sirtfoods means foods high in Sirtuins activators. Sirtuins help to protect the body cells from damaging, getting inflamed, and dying through sickness and disease. Scientific research has also proven that they also work to enhance the body muscle, regulate metabolic rate, and also burn fat.

Is Sirtfoods the Revolutionary Superfoods

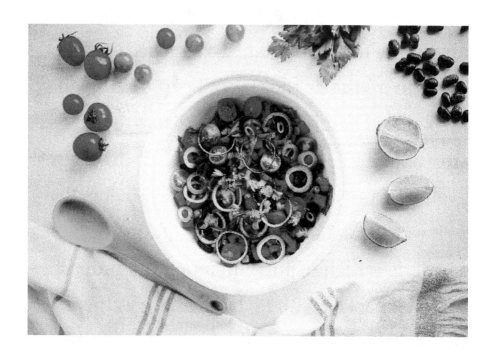

It's not a mere say that Sirtfoods is lovely and suitable for everyone. They are high in nutrients and packed with healthy compounds and properties. Few studies have been able to recommend that Sirtfoods have lots of healthy benefits. For instance, consuming the right amount of dark chocolate rich in cocoa content tends to minimize the risk of heart disease and help get rid of inflammation. Also, green tea is very potent in combating the risk of stroke and even all types of diabetes and likewise effective in lowering blood pressure. Additionally, turmeric is high in anti-inflammatory properties and well packed with high beneficiary effects on the body and can guide the body against all forms of health-related conditions. Most Sirtfoods have proven to have significant beneficiary effects in humans. There seems to be no concrete evidence on the beneficiary effects of an increased level of sirtuin proteins in humans. But particular research in cell lines and other animals has proven to be beneficial. For instance, an increase in the level of a certain Sirtuins protein level leads to prolonged lifespan in worms, yeast, and mice.

In the process of calorie restriction, sirtuin proteins notify the body to burn more fat to gain more energy and enhance insulin sensitivity. A particular study in mice stated that an increase in Sirtuins levels results in fat loss.

Other evidence also suggests that Sirtuins plays a vital role in minimizing inflammation, preventing the growth and development of tumours, and reducing the growth and development of heart-related disease and Alzheimer's.

Studies in humans and mice cell lines have indicated positive outcomes, but there are no human studies yet to state the impact that increased Sirtuins levels have on humans. Thus, there is no concrete evidence to ascertain that increment in Sirtuins protein levels in humans will bring about a prolonged lifespan or reduce the risk of cancer.

There's on-going research on the development of compounds that will be potent at increasing Sirtuins protein levels in the human body. Due to this, studies are continuing to know the impacts of Sirtuins in the human body.

Breakfast Recipes

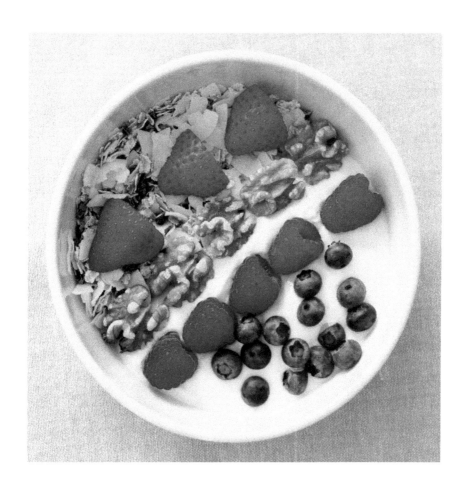

Strawberry Chocolate Shake

Preparation Time: *10 Minutes*

Cooking Time: *0 Minutes*

Servings: *1*

Ingredients:

1 cup water

1 cup frozen strawberries

1 oz baby arugula

½ avocado

½ teaspoon of vanilla extract

1 tablespoon of cacao powder

Directions

In a food processor, add in all the ingredients and blitz until smooth and creamy. Add ice for a thicker consistency, if desired. Serve immediately!

Nutrition: Calories 233, Fat: 7g, Carbs: 41g, Protein: 2g

Power Green Smoothie

Preparation Time: *10 minutes*

Cooking Time: *0 minutes*

Servings: *2*

Ingredients:

1 little gem lettuce, roughly chopped

2 cups almond milk

1 cup baby spinach, chopped

2 Medjool dates, pitted

A few ice cubes (optional)

Directions:

In a blender, mix in all the ingredients and pulse until completely smooth. Pour into two glasses and serve immediately.

Nutrition: Calories 114, Fat: 4g, Carbs: 23g, Protein: 2g

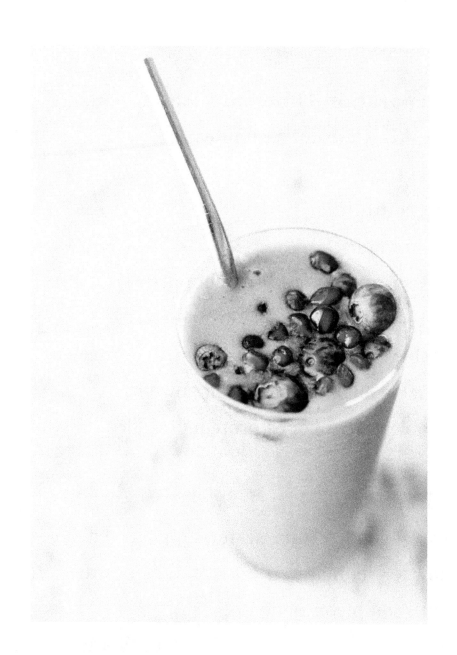

Energizing Cacao Protein Shake

Preparation Time: 10 minutes

Cooking Time: 0 minutes

Servings: 1

Ingredients:

1 cup water

1 green apple, cored and chopped

1 Medjool date, pitted

1 tablespoon of cacao powder

½ tablespoon of cinnamon powder

2 tablespoons of pea protein powder

4-5 ice cubes

Directions:

In a blender, mix water, apples, date, cacao powder, cinnamon, and protein powder. Blitz until completely smooth.

Add in the ice and pulse again until a thick and smooth texture is obtained. Serve right away!

Nutrition: Calories 253, Fat: 3g, Carbs: 49g, Protein: 15g

Morning Matcha Smoothie

Preparation Time: 10 minutes

Cooking Time: 0 minutes

Servings: 1

Ingredients:

1 cup almond milk

1 kiwi

½ avocado

½ inch fresh ginger, peeled (optional; add to taste)

1 handful of fresh baby spinach

½ teaspoon matcha powder

Directions:

In a blender, mix all ingredients and blitz until smooth. Add some pitted dates for more sweetness, if desired. Serve immediately!

Nutrition: Calories 316, Fat: 10g, Carbs: 61g, Protein: 8g

Ginger & Apple Green Smoothie

Preparation Time: 5 minutes

Cooking Time: 0 minutes

Servings: 2

Ingredients:

1 cup of cucumber, chopped

1 cup curly endive

1 apple, peeled and cored

2 tablespoons of lime juice

1 cups soy milk

½-inch piece peeled fresh ginger

1 tablespoon of chia seeds

1 cup unsweetened coconut yogurt

Directions:

Put in a food processor the cucumber, curly endive, apple, lime juice, soy milk, ginger, chia seeds, and coconut yogurt. Blend until smooth. Serve.

Nutrition*:* Calories 165, Fat*:* 4g, Carbs*:* 28g, Protein*:* 7g

Grilled Cauliflower Steaks

Preparation Time: *10 Minutes*

Cooking Time: *57 Minutes*

Servings: *4*

Ingredents:

2 medium heads cauliflower

2 medium shallots, peeled and minced

Water, as needed

1 clove garlic, peeled and minced

½ teaspoon ground fennel

½ teaspoon minced sage

½ teaspoon crushed red pepper flakes

½ cup green lentils, rinsed

2 cups of low-sodium vegetable broth

Salt, to taste (optional)

Freshly ground black pepper, to taste

Chopped parsley, for garnish

Directions:

On a flat work surface, cut each of the cauliflower heads in half through the stem, then trim each half, so you get a 1-inch-thick steak.

Arrange each piece on a baking sheet and set aside. You can reserve the extra cauliflower florets for other uses.

Sauté the shallots in a medium saucepan over medium heat for 10 minutes, stirring occasionally. Add water, 1 to 3 tablespoons at a time, to keep the shallots from sticking.

Stir in the garlic, fennel, sage, red pepper flakes, and lentils and cook for 3 minutes.

Pour into the vegetable broth and bring to a boil over high heat.

Grill the cauliflower steaks for about 7 minutes per side until evenly browned.

Transfer the cauliflower steaks to a plate and spoon the purée over them. Serve garnished with the parsley.

Nutrition: Calories: 105, Fat: 1g, Carbs: 18g, Protein: 5g

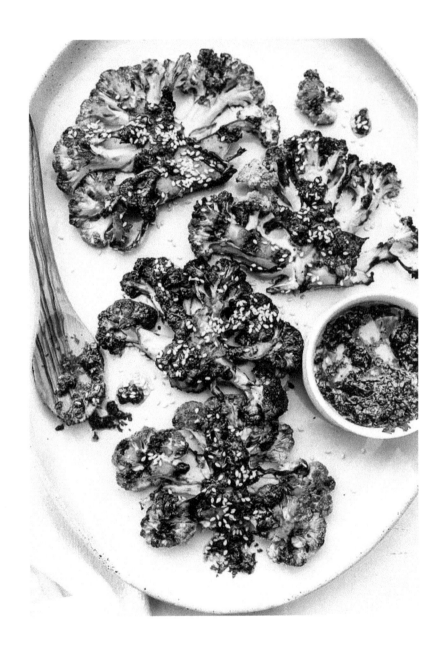

Treacle Buckwheat Granola

Preparation Time: 15 minutes

Cooking Time: 0 minutes

Servings: 1

Ingredients:

1 cup buckwheat groats

½ cup chopped pecans

½ cup shredded coconut

1 tablespoon of chia seeds

1 tablespoon of date sugar

A pinch of sea salt

½ teaspoon of ground cardamom

½ cup olive oil

½ cup black treacle (or molasses)

Directions:

Preheat oven to 320 F. In a bowl, add the all the ingredients and stir to combine.

In a small saucepan over medium-low heat, warm the oil and black treacle until melted and well combined. Spread the mixture evenly onto a lined baking sheet and bake for 25-30 minutes, stirring halfway through for an even baking.

Nutrition: Calories 270, Fat: 8g, Carbs: 52g, Protein: 9g

Cinnamon Buckwheat with Walnuts

Preparation Time: 10 minutes

Cooking Time: 20 minutes

Servings: 1

Ingredients:

1 cup of almond milk

1 cup of water

1 cup of buckwheat groats, rinsed

1 teaspoon of cinnamon

¼ cup of walnuts, chopped

2 tablespoon of pure date syrup

Directions:

Place almond milk, water, and buckwheat in a pot over medium heat. Lower the heat and simmer covered for 15 minutes. Allow sitting covered for 5 minutes. Mix in the cinnamon, walnuts, and date syrup. Serve warm.

Nutrition: Calories 245, Fat*:* 9g, Carbs*:* 37g, Protein*:* 7g

Instant Savoury Gigante Beans

Preparation Time: *10-30 Minutes*

Cooking Time: *55 Minutes*

Servings: *6*

Ingredients:

1 lb. Gigante Beans, soaked overnight

½ cup of olive oil

1 onion, sliced

2 cloves garlic, crushed or minced

1 red bell pepper, cut into ⅓ inch pieces

2 carrots, sliced

½ teaspoon of salt and ground black pepper

2 tomatoes peeled, grated

1 tablespoon of celery, chopped

1 tablespoon of tomato paste (or ketchup)

¾ teaspoon of sweet paprika

1 teaspoon of oregano

1 cup vegetable broth

Directions:

Soak Gigante beans overnight.

Press the SAUTÉ button on your Instant Pot and heat the oil.

Sauté onion, garlic, sweet pepper, carrots with a pinch of salt for 3 - 4 minutes; stir occasionally.

Add rinsed Gigante beans into your Instant Pot along with all remaining ingredients and stir well.

Latch lid into place and set on the MANUAL setting for 25 minutes.

When the beep sounds, quick release the pressure by pressing Cancel and twisting the steam handle to the Venting position.

Taste and adjust seasonings to taste.

Serve warm or cold.

Keep refrigerated.

Nutrition: Calories 502, Fat: 6g, Carbs: 31g, Protein: 9g

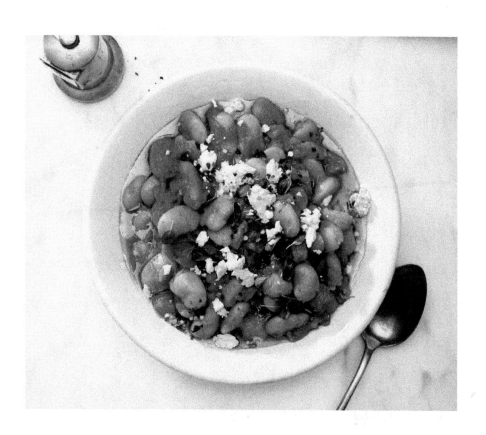

Instant Turmeric Risotto

Preparation Time: *10-30 Minutes*

Cooking Time: *40 Minutes*

Servings: *4*

Ingredents:

4 tablespoons of olive oil

1 cup of onion

1 teaspoon of minced garlic

2 cups of long-grain rice

3 cups of vegetable broth

½ teaspoon of paprika (smoked)

½ teaspoon of turmeric

½ teaspoon of nutmeg

2 Tablespoon of fresh basil leaves chopped

Salt and ground black pepper to taste

Directions:

Press the SAUTÉ button on your Instant Pot and heat oil.

Sauté the onion and garlic with a pinch of salt until softened.

Add the rice and all leftover ingredients and stir well.

Lock the lid into place and set on and select the RICE button for 10 minutes.

Press Cancel when the timer beeps and carefully flip the Quick Release valve to let the pressure out.

Taste and adjust seasonings to taste.

Serve.

Nutrition: Calories 559, Fat: 6g, Carbs: 29g, Protein: 9g

Nettle Soup with Rice

Preparation Time: *10-30 Minutes*

Cooking Time: *40 Minutes*

Servings: *5*

Ingredents:

3 tablespoons of of olive oil

2 onions, finely chopped

2 cloves garlic, finely chopped

Salt and freshly ground black pepper

4 medium potatoes, cut into cubes

1 cup of rice

1 tablespoon of arrowroot

2 cups of vegetable broth

2 cups of water

1 bunch of young nettle leaves packed

½ cup fresh parsley, finely chopped

1 teaspoon of cumin

Directions:

Heat olive oil in a large pot.

Sauté onion and garlic with a pinch of salt until softened.

Add potato, rice, and arrowroot; sauté for 2 to 3 minutes.

Pour broth and water, stir well, cover and cook over medium heat for about 20 minutes.

Cook for about 30 to 45 minutes.

Add young nettle leaves, parsley, and cumin; stir and cook for 5 to 7 minutes.

Move the soup in a blender and blend until combined well.

Taste and adjust salt and pepper.

Serve hot.

Nutrition: Calories 421, Fat: 8g, Carbs: 18g, Protein: 10g

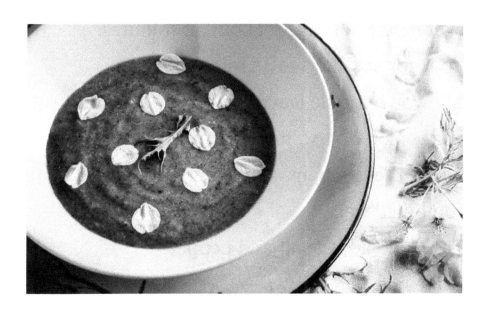

Okra with Grated Tomatoes

Preparation Time: *10-30 Minutes*

Cooking Time: 3 Hours and 10 Minutes

Servings: *4*

Ingredients:

2 lbs. fresh okra, cleaned

2 onions, finely chopped

2 cloves garlic, finely sliced

2 carrots, sliced

2 ripe tomatoes, grated

1 cup of water

4 tablespoon of olive oil

Salt and ground black pepper

1 tablespoon of fresh parsley, finely chopped

Directions:

Add okra in your Crock-Pot: sprinkle with a pinch of salt and pepper. Add in chopped onion, garlic, carrots, and grated tomatoes; stir well. Pour water and oil, season with the salt, pepper, and give a good stir.

Covering and cook on LOW for 2-4 hours or until tender.

Open the lid and add fresh parsley; stir. Taste and adjust salt and pepper.

Serve hot.

Nutrition: Calories 249, Fat: 8g, Carbs: 21g, Protein: 8g

Oven-Baked Smoked Lentil Burgers

Preparation Time: *10-30 Minutes*

Cooking Time: 1 Hour and 20 Minutes

Servings: 6

Ingredents:

1 ½ cups of dried lentils

3 cups of water

Salt and ground black pepper to taste

2 tablespoons of olive oil

1 onion, finely diced

2 cloves of garlic, minced

1 cup of button mushrooms sliced

2 tablespoons of tomato paste

½ teaspoon of fresh basil, finely chopped

1 cup of chopped almonds

3 teaspoon of balsamic vinegar

3 tablespoon of coconut amino

1 teaspoon of liquid smoke

¾ cup silken tofu soft

¾ cup corn starch

Directions:

Cook lentils in salted water until tender or for about 30-35 minutes; rinse, drain, and set aside.

Heat oil in a frying skillet and sauté onion, garlic, and mushrooms for 4 to 5 minutes; stir occasionally.

Stir in the tomato paste, salt, basil, salt, and black pepper; cook for 2 to 3 minutes.

Stir in almonds, vinegar, coconut amino, liquid smoke, and lentils.

Remove from heat and stir in blended tofu and corn starch.

Keep stirring until all ingredients combined well.

Form mixture into patties and refrigerate for an hour.

Preheat oven to 350 F.

Line a baking dish with parchment paper and arrange patties on the pan.

Bake for 20 to 25 minutes.

Serve hot with buns, green salad, tomato sauce, etc.

Nutrition: Calories 532, Fat: 7g, Carbs: 20g, Protein: 6g

Powerful Spinach and Mustard Leaves Puree

Preparation Time: *10-30 Minutes*

Cooking Time: *50 Minutes*

Servings: *4*

Ingredients:

2 Tablespoon of almond butter

One onion finely diced

2 Tablespoon of minced garlic

1 teaspoon of salt and black pepper (or to taste)

1 lb. mustard leaves cleaned rinsed

1 lb. frozen spinach thawed

1 teaspoon of coriander

1 teaspoon of ground cumin

½ cup almond milk

Directions:

Press the SAUTÉ button on your Instant Pot and heat the almond butter. Sauté onion, garlic, and a pinch of salt for 2-3 minutes; stir occasionally.

Add spinach and the mustard greens and stir for a minute or two. Season with the salt and pepper, coriander, and cumin; give a good stir.

Lock lid into place and set on the MANUAL setting for 15 minutes.

Use Quick Release - turn the valve from sealing to venting to release the pressure.

Move mixture to a blender, add almond milk and blend until smooth.

Taste and adjust seasonings. Serve.

Nutrition: Calories 290, Fat: 6g, Carbs: 26g, Protein: 9g

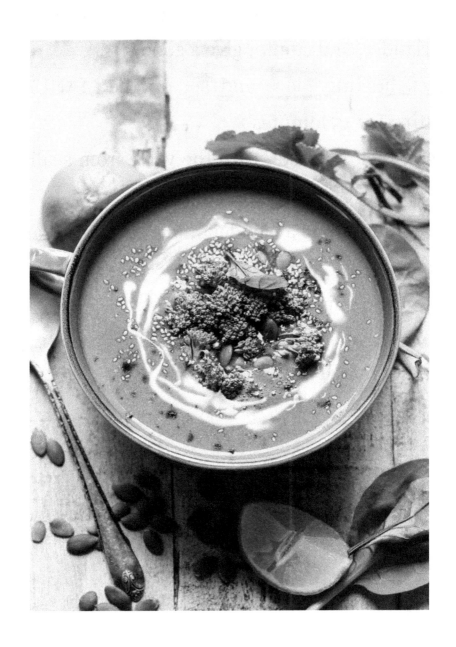

Moroccan Spiced Eggs

Preparation time: 1 hour 10 minutes

Cooking time: 45 minutes

Servings: 2

Ingredients:

1 tablespoon olive oil

1 shallot, stripped and finely hacked

1 red (chime) pepper, deseeded and finely hacked

1 garlic clove, stripped and finely hacked

1 courgette (zucchini), stripped and finely hacked

1 tablespoon tomato puree (glue)

½ teaspoon gentle stew powder

¼ teaspoon ground cinnamon

¼ teaspoon ground cumin

½ teaspoon salt

400g can hacked tomatoes

400g may chickpeas in water

A little bunch of level leaf parsley cleaved

4 medium eggs at room temperature

Directions:

Heat the oil in a pan, include the shallot and red (ringer) pepper and fry delicately for 5 minutes. At that point include the garlic and courgette (zucchini) and cook for one more moment or two. Include the tomato puree (glue), flavors and salt and mix through.

Add the cleaved tomatoes and chickpeas (dousing alcohol and all) and increment the warmth to medium. With the top of the dish, stew the sauce for 30 minutes – ensure it is delicately rising all through and permit it to lessen in volume by around 33%.

Remove from the warmth and mix in the cleaved parsley.

Preheat the grill to 200C/180C fan/350F.

When you are prepared to cook the eggs, bring the tomato sauce up to a delicate stew and move to a little broiler confirmation dish.

Crack the eggs on the dish and lower them delicately into the stew. Spread with thwart and prepare in the grill for 10-15 minutes. Serve the blend in unique dishes with the eggs coasting on the top.

Nutrition: Calories 112, Fat: 5g, Carbs: 13g, Protein: 6g

Sirt Chili Con Carne

Preparation time: 1 hour 20 minutes

Cooking time: 1 hour 3 minutes

Servings: 4

Ingredients:

1 red onion, finely cleaved

3 garlic cloves, finely cleaved

2 10,000 foot chilies, finely hacked

1 tablespoon additional virgin olive oil

1 tablespoon ground cumin

1 tablespoon ground turmeric

400g lean minced hamburger (5 percent fat)

150ml red wine

1 red pepper, cored, seeds evacuated and cut into reduced down pieces

2 x 400g tins cleaved tomatoes

1 tablespoon tomato purée

1 tablespoon cocoa powder

300ml hamburger stock

5g coriander, cleaved

5g parsley, cleaved

160g buckwheat

Directions:

In a meal, fry the onion, garlic and bean stew in the oil over a medium heat for 2-3 minutes, at that point include the flavors and cook for a moment.

Include the minced hamburger and dark colored over a high heat. Include the red wine and permit it to rise to decrease it considerably.

You may need to add a little water to accomplish a thick, clingy consistency. Just before serving, mix in the hacked herbs.

In the interim, cook the buckwheat as indicated by the bundle guidelines and present with the stew.

Nutrition: Calories 342, Fat: 11g, Carbs: 29g, Protein: 14g

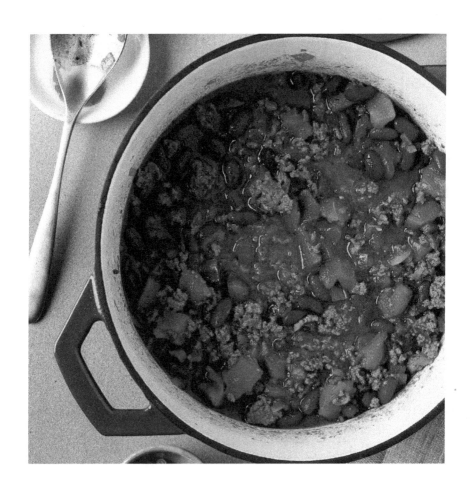

Salmon and Spinach Quiche

Preparation time: 55 minutes

Cooking time: 45 minutes

Servings: 2

Ingredients:

600g frozen leaf spinach

1 clove of garlic

1 onion

150g frozen salmon fillets

200g smoked salmon

1 small Bunch of dill

1 untreated lemon

50 g butter

200 g sour cream

3 eggs

Salt, pepper, nutmeg

1 pack of puff pastry

Directions:

Let the spinach thaw and squeeze well.

Peel the garlic and onion and cut into fine cubes.

Cut the salmon fillet into cubes 1-1.5 cm thick.

Cut the smoked salmon into strips.

Wash the dill, pat dry and chop.

Wash the lemon with hot water, dry, rub the zest finely with a kitchen grater and squeeze the lemon.

Heat the butter in a pan. Sweat the garlic and onion cubes in it for approx. 2-3 minutes.

Add spinach and sweat briefly.

Add sour cream, lemon juice and zest, eggs and dill and mix well.

Season with salt, pepper and nutmeg.

Preheat the oven to 200 degrees' top / bottom heat (180 degrees' convection).

Grease a spring form pan and roll out the puff pastry in it and pull up on edge. Prick the dough with a fork (so that it doesn't rise too much).

Pour in the spinach and egg mixture and smooth out.

Spread salmon cubes and smoked salmon strips on top.

The quiche in the oven (grid, middle inset) about 30-40 min. Yellow gold bake.

Nutrition: Calories 320, Fat: 8g, Carbs: 18g, Protein: 12g

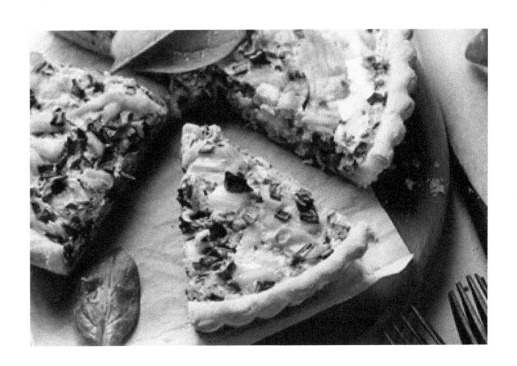

Choc Chip Granola

Preparation time: 55 minutes

Cooking time: 20 minutes

Servings: 2

Ingredients:

200g large oat flakes

Roughly 50 g pecan nuts chopped

3 tablespoons of light olive oil

20g butter

1 tablespoon of dark brown sugar

2 tablespoon rice syrup

60 g of good quality (70%)

Dark chocolate shavings

Directions:

Oven preheats to 160 ° C (140 ° C fan / Gas 3).
Line a large baking tray with a sheet of silicone or
parchment for baking.

In a large bowl, combine the oats and pecans. Heat the olive oil, butter, brown sugar, and rice malt syrup gently in a small non-stick pan until the butter has melted, and the sugar and syrup dissolve. Do not let boil. Pour the syrup over the oats and stir thoroughly until fully covered with the oats.

Spread the granola over the baking tray and spread right into the corners. Leave the mixture clumps with spacing, instead of even spreading. Bake for 20 minutes in the oven until golden brown is just tinged at the edges. Remove from the oven, and leave completely to cool on the tray.

When cold, split with your fingers any larger lumps on the tray and then mix them in the chocolate chips. Put the granola in an airtight tub or jar, or pour it. The granola is to last for at least 2 weeks.

Nutrition: Calories 521, Fat: 6g, Carbs: 29g, Protein: 18g

Kale & Red Onion Salsa

Preparation time: 55 minutes

Cooking time: 30 minutes

Servings: 2

Ingredients:

Chicken breast

2 teaspoons ground turmeric

Lemon

Olive oil

Kale

Red onion

Ginger

Buckwheat

Directions:

Add the chili, parsley, capers, lemon juice and mix.

Preheat the oven to 220°C. Pour 1 teaspoon of the turmeric, the lemon juice and a little oil on the chicken breast and marinate. Allow to stay for 5–10 minutes.

Place an ovenproof frying pan on the heat and cook the marinated chicken for a minute on each side to achieve a pale golden color. Then transfer the pan containing the chicken to the oven and allow to stay for 8–10 minutes or until it is done. Remove from the oven and cover with foil, set aside for 5 minutes before serving.

Put the kale in a steamer and cook for 5 minutes. Pour a little oil in a frying pan and fry the red onions and the ginger to become soft but not coloured. Add the cooked kale and continue to fry for another minute.

Cook the buckwheat following the packet's instructions using the remaining turmeric. Serve alongside the chicken, salsa, and vegetables.

Nutrition: Calories 129, Fat: 8g, Carbs: 19g, Protein: 9g

Leek with Pine Nuts

Preparation time: 45 minutes

Cooking time: 15 minutes

Servings: 2

Ingredients:

20g Ghee

2 teaspoon Olive oil

2 pieces Leek

150 ml Vegetable broth

Fresh parsley

1 tablespoon fresh oregano

1 tablespoon Pine nuts (roasted)

Directions:

Cook the leek until golden brown for 5 minutes, stirring constantly.

Add the vegetable broth and cook for another 10 minutes until the leek is tender.

Stir in the herbs and sprinkle the pine nuts on the dish just before serving.

Nutrition: Calories 158, Fat: 6g, Carbs: 17g, Protein: 9g

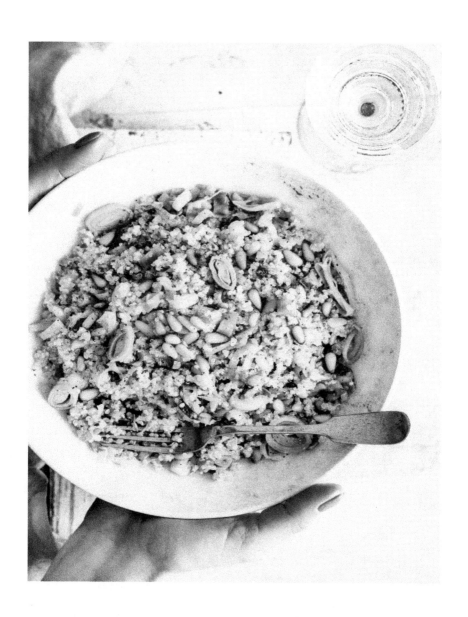

Lunch Recipes

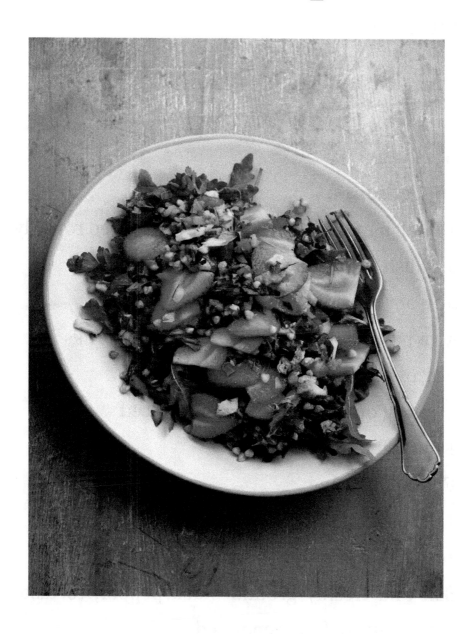

Salmon salad with mint dressing

Preparation time: 5 minutes

Cooking time: 30 minutes

Servings: 3

Ingredients:

1 small handful (10g) of parsley, chopped roughly

2 radishes, trimmed and thinly sliced

40g of young spinach leaves

5cm piece (50g) cucumber, cut into chunks

40g of mixed salad leaves

2 spring onions, trimmed then sliced

1 salmon fillet (130g)

For the dressing:

1 tablespoon of of rice vinegar

1 teaspoon of of low-fat mayonnaise

Salt and freshly ground black pepper, to taste

2mint leaves, finely chopped

1 tablespoon of of natural yoghurt

Directions:

Preheat your oven to 200 degrees. Place salmon fillets on a baking tray and allow them to bake for about 16-18 minutes.

Remove from the oven and then let them rest (salmon is ok served hot or cold when added to the salad).

Remove the skin of your salmon (if it has one) after cooking.

Mix the mayonnaise, mint leaves, rice wine vinegar, salt, yoghurt, and pepper in a small bowl and let it stand for 5 minutes to let the flavour deepen.

Place the salad leaves with the spinach on top of a plate and top with the radishes, spring onions, cucumber, and parsley.

Flake the salmon onto the salad then drizzle the dressing over.

Nutrition: Calories 245, Fat: 2g, Carbs: 10g, Protein: 3g

Hearty quinoa and spinach breakfast casserole

Preparation time: 5 minutes

Cooking time: 20 minutes

Servings: 3

Ingredients:

1 cup cooked quinoa

3-4 spring onions, finely chopped

5 oz frozen chopped spinach, thawed and squeezed dry

½ zucchini, peeled and shredded

5 eggs

½ cup milk

4 tablespoon of extra virgin olive oil

salt and black pepper, to taste

1 cup cheddar cheese, grated

Directions:

In a large bowl combine eggs, milk, salt and pepper.

In a deep casserole dish heat, the olive oil.

Cook the onions, zucchini and spinach, stirring constantly, until lightly cooked.

Add in the quinoa and combine everything well.

Pour the egg mixture over and then top with cheddar cheese.

Bake in a preheated to 350 f oven for 20 minutes.

Nutrition: Calories 211, Fat: 2g, Carbs: 10g, Protein: 2g

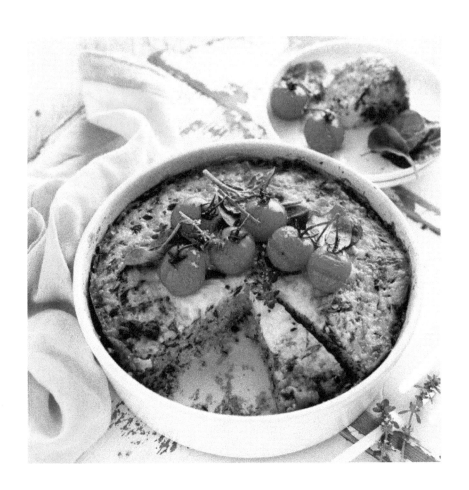

Quick quinoa vegetable scramble

Preparation time: 5 minutes

Cooking time: 30 minutes

Servings: 3

Ingredients:

½ cup cooked quinoa

½ small onion, chopped

2 tomatoes, diced

1 large red pepper, chopped

5 eggs

½ cup crumbled feta

4 tablespoon of extra virgin olive oil

Black pepper, to taste

Salt, to taste

Directions:

In a large pan, sauté onion over medium heat for 1-2 minutes, stirring.

Add in tomatoes and red pepper and cook until the mixture is almost dry.

Stir in quinoa, feta and eggs and cook until well mixed and not too liquid.

Season with black pepper and serve.

Nutrition: Calories 234, Fat: 2g, Carbs: 19g, Protein: 3g

Coconut and quinoa banana pudding

Preparation time: 5 minutes
Cooking time: 30 minutes
Servings: 3

Ingredients:

1 cup quinoa

3 cups coconut milk

3 ripe bananas

¼ cup flaked unsweetened coconut

4 tablespoon of sugar

1 teaspoon of vanilla extract

Directions:

Wash and cook quinoa according to package directions.

When ready remove from heat and set aside.

In a separate bowl blend sugar, milk and bananas until smooth.

Add to the quinoa.

Heat over medium heat, string, until creamy.

Stir in vanilla and coconut flakes and serve warm.

Nutrition: Calories 211, Fat: 3g, Carbs: 12g, Protein: 9g

Chicken with kale and chilli salsa

Preparation time: 5 minutes

Cooking time: 40 minutes

Servings: 3

Ingredients:

50g of buckwheat

1 teaspoon of of chopped fresh ginger

Juice of ½ lemon, divided

Turmeric

Kale

Onion

Olive oil

Tomato

Parsley

Chilli

Directions:

Start with the salsa: remove the eye out of the tomato and finely chop it, making sure to keep as much of the liquid as you can.

Mix it with the chilli, parsley, and lemon juice.

You could add everything to a blender for different results.

Heat your oven to 220F.

Marinate the chicken with a little oil, 1 teaspoon of of turmeric, and the lemon juice.

Let it rest for 5-10 minutes.

Heat a pan over medium heat until it is hot then add marinated chicken and allow it to cook for a minute on both sides until it is pale gold).

Transfer the chicken to the oven (if pan is not ovenproof place it in a baking tray) and bake for 8 to 10 minutes or until it is cooked through.

Take the chicken out of the oven, cover with foil, and let it rest for five minutes before you serve.

Meanwhile, in a steamer, steam the kale for about 5 minutes.

In a little oil, fry the ginger and red onions until they are soft but not coloured, and then add in the cooked kale and fry it for a minute.

Cook the buckwheat in accordance to the packet directions with the remainig turmeric.

Serve alongside the vegetables, salsa and chicken.

Nutrition: Calories 213, Fat: 6g, Carbs: 7g, Protein: 22g

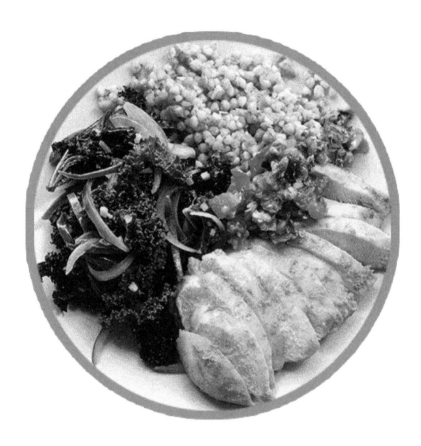

Sirt salmon salad

Preparation time: 5 minutes

Cooking time: 30 minutes

Servings: 3

Ingredients:

1 large Medjool date, pitted then chopped

Olive oil

Parsley

Celery leaves

Walnuts

Capers

Red onions-sliced

Smoked salmon slices

Directions:

Arrange all the salad leaves on a large plate then mix the rest of the ingredients and distribute evenly on top the leaves.

Nutrition: Calories 453, Fat: 4g, Carbs: 8g, Protein: 19g

Greek salad skewers

Preparation time: 5 minutes

Cooking time: 30 minutes

Servings: 3

Ingredients:

Cucumber

Tomatoes

 Black olives

Red onion

Skewers

   For the dressing:

Juice of ½ lemon

½ garlic clove, peeled and crushed

1 tablespoon of of extra virgin olive oil

A few leaves of finely chopped basil

Generous seasoning of salt and freshly ground black pepper a few finely chopped oregano leaves

1 teaspoon of of balsamic vinegar

Directions:

Thread every skewer with salad ingredients in this order; olive, followed by tomato, then yellow pepper, red onion, followed by cucumber then feta, tomato, olive, then yellow pepper, red onion and finally cucumber.

Place the dressing ingredients in a small bowl, mix them thoroughly, and then pour over the skewers.

Nutrition: Calories 209, Fat: 8g, Carbs: 8g, Protein: 21g

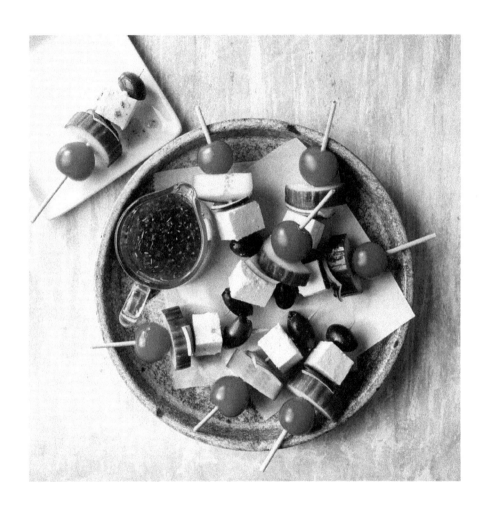

Mediterranean Chicken Breasts

Preparation time: 5 minutes

Cooking time: 1 hour 5 minutes

Servings: 2

Ingredients:

2 teaspoon of olive oil

1 medium lemon, sliced

½ lb chicken breasts, halved

Salt and black pepper to season

1 tablespoon of capers, rinsed

1 cup chicken broth

2 tablespoons of chopped fresh parsley, divided

Directions:

Lay a piece of parchment paper on a baking sheet. Preheat the oven to 350°F.

Lay the lemon slices on the baking sheet, drizzle them with olive oil and sprinkle with salt. Roast in the oven for 25 minutes to brown the lemon rinds.

Cover the chicken with plastic wrap, place them on a flat surface, and gently pound with the rolling pin to flatten to about ½ -inch thickness.

Remove the plastic wraps and season the chicken with salt and pepper; set aside.

Heat the olive oil in a skillet over medium heat and fry the chicken on both sides to a golden brown for about 8 minutes in total.

Then, pour the chicken broth in, shake the skillet, and let the broth boil and reduce to a thick consistency, about 12 minutes.

Lightly stir in capers, roasted lemon, black pepper, olive oil, and parsley; simmer on low heat for 10 minutes. Serve the chicken with the sauce and sprinkled with fresh parsley.

Nutrition: Calories 430, Fat: 23g, Carbs: 13g, Protein: 33g

Greek-Style Chicken with Olives & Capers

Preparation time: 5 minutes

Cooking time: 20 minutes

Servings: 2

Ingredients:

1 red onion, chopped

½ lb chicken breasts, skinless and boneless

2 garlic cloves, minced

1 tablespoon of capers

2 tomatoes, chopped

½ teaspoon of red chili flakes

Directions: Warm olive oil in a skillet over medium heat and cook the chicken for 2 minutes per side. Sprinkle with black pepper and salt. Set the chicken breasts in the oven at 450°F and bake for 8 minutes. Arrange the chicken on a platter.

In the same pan over medium heat, add the onion, olives, capers, garlic, and chili flakes, and cook for 1 minute. Stir in the tomatoes, pepper, and salt, and cook for 2 minutes. Sprinkle over the chicken breasts and enjoy.

Nutrition: Calories 387, Fat: 21g, Carbs: 12g, Protein: 23g

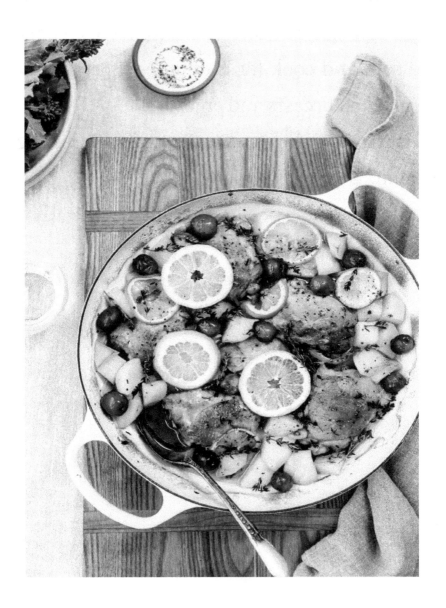

Fried Cod with Celery Wine Sauce

Preparation time: 5 minutes
Cooking time: 15 minutes

Servings: 2

Ingredients:

2 teaspoon of extra-virgin olive oil

2 cod fillets

2 garlic cloves, minced

Juice of 1 lemon

3 tablespoon of white wine

1 stalk celery, chopped

1 small red onion, chopped

Salt and black pepper to taste

Directions:

Heat 2 tablespoon of of the oil in a skillet over medium heat and season the cod with salt and black pepper. Fry the fillets in the oil for 4 minutes on one side, flip and cook for 1 minute. Take out, plate, and set aside.

In another skillet over low heat, warm the remaining olive oil and sauté the garlic and celery for 3 minutes. Add the lemon juice, wine, and red onions. Season with salt, black pepper, and cook for 3 minutes until the wine slightly reduces.

Put the fish in the skillet, spoon sauce over, cook for 30 seconds, and turn the heat off. Divide fish into plates, top with sauce, and serve.

Nutrition: Calories 264, Fat: 17g, Carbs: 9g, Protein: 20g

Minty Pesto Rubbed Beef Tenderloins

Preparation time: 5 minutes

Cooking time: 3 hours 10 minutes

Servings: 1

Ingredients:

1 cup fresh parsley, roughly chopped

1 teaspoon of fresh mint

1 red onion, chopped

5 oz beef tenderloin

1 lemon zested and juiced

3 tablespoon of olive oil, divided

1 oz walnuts, chopped

Salt to taste

3 garlic cloves, minced

Directions:

Preheat oven to 360 F.

In a food processor, combine the parsley with 2 tablespoons of of olive oil, mint, garlic, walnuts, salt, lemon zest, and red onion. Rub the beef with the mixture, place in a bowl, and refrigerate for 1 hour covered.

Remove the beef and warm 1 tablespoon of of olive oil in a skillet over high heat. Sear the meat for 3 to 5 minutes, depending on how you like it done. Transfer to a baking dish and cook in the oven for 16 minutes. Serve with a salad.

Nutrition: Calories 528, Fat: 38g, Carbs: 23g, Protein: 37g

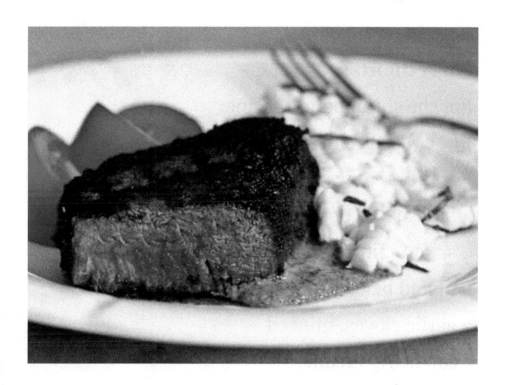

Crispy Salmon Shirataki Fettucine

Preparation time: 5 minutes

Cooking time: 30 minutes

Servings: 2

Ingredients:

For the shirataki fettuccine:

1 (4 oz) pack shirataki fettuccine

For the creamy salmon sauce:

3 tablespoon of extra-virgin olive oil

2 salmon fillets, cut into 2-inch cubes

Salt and black pepper to taste

3 garlic cloves, minced

1 cup heavy cream

½ cup dry white wine

1 teaspoon of grated lemon zest

1 cup baby spinach

Lemon wedges for garnishing

Directions:

For the shirataki fettuccine:

Boil 2 cups of water in a pot over medium heat. Strain the shirataki pasta through a colander and rinse very well under hot running water. Pour the shirataki pasta into the boiling water. Take off the heat, let sit for 3 minutes and strain again.

Place a dry skillet over medium heat and stir-fry the shirataki pasta until visibly dry, and makes a squeaky sound when stirred, 1 to 2 minutes. Take off the heat and set aside.

For the salmon sauce:

Melt half of the olive oil in a large skillet; season the salmon with salt, black pepper, and cook in the butter until golden brown on all sides and flaky within, 8 minutes. Transfer to a plate and set aside. Add the remaining olive oil to the skillet and stir in the garlic. Cook until fragrant, 1 minute.

Mix in heavy cream, white wine, lemon zest, salt, and pepper. Allow boiling over low heat for 5 minutes. Stir in spinach, allow wilting for 2 minutes and stir in shirataki fettuccine and salmon until well-coated in the sauce. Garnish with the lemon wedges.

Nutrition: Calories 473, Fat: 48g, Carbs: 21g, Protein: 25g

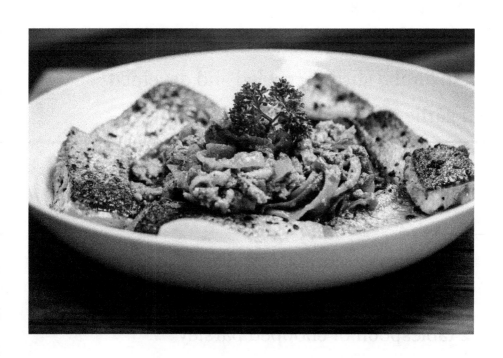

Parsley-Lime Shrimp Pasta

Preparation time: 5 minutes

Cooking time: 15 minutes

Servings: 4

Ingredients:

2 tablespoon of butter

1 lb jumbo shrimp, peeled and deveined

4 garlic cloves, minced

1 pinch red chili flakes

¼ cup white wine

1 lime, zested and juiced

3 medium zucchinis, spiralized

Salt and black pepper to taste

2 tablespoon of chopped parsley

1 cup grated Parmesan cheese for topping

Directions:

Melt the butter in a large skillet and cook the shrimp until starting to turn pink.

Flip and stir in the garlic and red chili flakes. Cook further for 1 minute or until the shrimp is pink and opaque. Transfer to a plate and set aside.

Pour the wine and lime juice into the skillet, and cook until reduced by a quarter. Meanwhile, stir to deglaze the bottom of the pot.

Mix in the zucchinis, lime zest, shrimp, and parsley. Season with salt and black pepper, and toss everything well. Cook until the zucchinis is slightly tender for 2 minutes. Dish the food onto serving plates and top generously with the Parmesan cheese.

Nutrition: Calories 315, Fat: 10g, Carbs: 43g, Protein: 27g

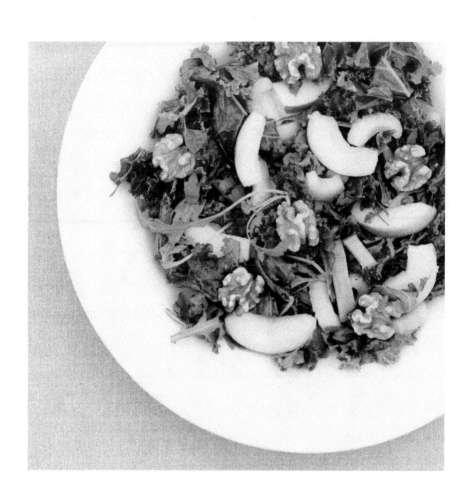

CPSIA information can be obtained
at www.ICGtesting.com
Printed in the USA
BVHW010424130321
602399BV00005B/247